School Girls Rock

School Girls Rock

*Curriculum and Guide to
Educational Achievement*

Dr. Andrea Green-Gibson

Library of Congress Control Number:		2013915961
ISBN:	Hardcover	978-1-4836-9467-2
	Softcover	978-1-4836-9466-5
	Ebook	978-1-4836-9468-9

This book was printed in the United States of America.

Rev. date: 11/13/2013

To order additional copies of this book, contact:
Xlibris LLC
1-888-795-4274
www.Xlibris.com
Orders@Xlibris.com
135615

Contents

Contents

Dedication

I dedicate this book to all Chicago Public Schools (CPS) students and educators as well as all parents/guardians of students who attend CPS. A plethora of our nation's youth particularly, female-youth and their parents/guardians and teachers work extremely hard to reach set goals and achieve academic success. Often times, ineffective circumstances affect the academic success rates producing undesirable outcomes for each group involved in the learning and schooling processes. This book is dedicated to the leaders and those whom wield the power to make meaningful yet, effective change to the field of education, particularly, public education for African-American, female students.

Introduction

IN THE 21ST century, the majority of our nation's youth are still performing below standards in many public schools. The notion is that, *education in the key to success* but it seems the terms "education" and "schooling" should be examined using several lenses particularly, in Chicago Public Schools (CPS). When speaking about education and schooling, both processes are directly related to culture, according to researchers who purported, "the deliberate transmission of culture is called **education**" and "The formal and more restrictive process of cultural transmission may be called **schooling**" (Pai & Adler, 2001). Nobles (1990) stated the following:

> Technically, culture is the vast structure of behaviors, ideas, attitudes, values, habits, beliefs, customs, language, rituals, ceremonies, and practices peculiar to a particular group of people which provides them with a general design for living and patterns for interpreting reality. The system of culture teaches the people to recognize phenomenon and to respect certain logical relations amongst phenomena. Culture gives meaning to reality. As such, culture has the power to compel behavior and the capacity to reinforce ideas and beliefs about human functioning, including issues of educational achievement and motivation. As such, culture is the invisible **medium** in which all human functioning occurs. It is important to note, in fact, that nothing human

happens outside of culture. To think of culture as the medium in the Petrie dish is an appropriate analogy. It is the stuff in which human development occurs. Culture is to humans like water is to fish. It is our total environment. As such, education as well as curriculum development is cultural phenomenon. Culture is therefore the invisible dimension of all curricula. (p. 6).

Culture being a major factor in educational development, the team at **School Girls Rock (SGR)** will work to tailor culture towards attending student's needs. A growing body of researchers reported that educational leaders are constantly searching to find the best methods for teaching African-American students who attend urban public schools (NCLB, 2002). Educational leaders from the SGR program are beginning to explore the possibility that infusing etiquette and nutrition in the schooling process may help African-American female students learn more effectively.

SGR is powered by ShaDavAli Multimedia Studio Inc., (SMSI). A specialized program designed to help improve the quality of education for our nation's female-youth by fostering mentorship and infusing etiquettes as well as nutrition in the curriculum. The SGR group leaders will provide guidance to students that will enable better performance in regular education classrooms, at home, and in the community. Encouraging girls to believe that dreams come true with hard work and determination; set goals; aim high; and challenge their abilities, is the purpose of the SGR program. Group leaders at SGR have developed an approach that will work to foster the purpose by infusing etiquettes and nutrition in the curriculum. There is a relationship between what one eats and how one behaves, which has an effect on the value of one's livelihood. From the SGR program, students will:

1. Gain a sense of pride, self-confidence, and awareness;
2. Understand how to work in cohorts, effectively;

3. Learn to reveal her persona appropriately with respect to self, parents, peers, the elderly, and other individuals;
4. Learn the benefits of healthy eating habits;
5. Understand and value her inner and outer beauty as well as that of her peers and elder, and
6. Encounter a sense of balance: Your body is your temple, embrace it!

Girls of diverse cultural backgrounds are welcome to join the SGR program and each personality will be explored, as a means to provide a meaningful learning experience for all SGR members. Each girl will have a membership or "royal" number, which represents fellowship and wear a SGR specialized badge of honor.

☑ Royal Number—A number is assigned to each girl in the order of enrollment starting with 101. Each girl will learn that she is indigenous of royalty then provided her royal number.

☑ Badge of Honor—A badge that represents SGR membership and is worn in honor of young girls who seek encouragement, academic success, and valuable endeavors at home, in their community, and the world.

Background of Public School System

IN THE EARLY 1960s, African-Americans petitioned for full civil rights including equal educational opportunities (Pai & Adler, 2001) and insisted that their cultural patterns exist and develop in their own way (Carruthers, 1995; Marks & Tonso, 2006; Pai & Adler, 2001; Shujaa, 1996, 1998). As a result, according to Pai and Adler, President Lyndon B. Johnson introduced the Great Society programs, which included educational measures such as the *Economic Opportunity Act of 1964* and the *Elementary and Secondary Education Act of 1965*. The idea of the Great Society programs was for America to become a society in which all groups have parity in power (Pai & Adler). Social, political, and economic equality was to be achieved by providing equal educational opportunities for all races of people (Pai & Adler). Compensatory education is a significant part of the Great Society programs according to Pai and Adler (2001) who stated that the purpose was to lift African-Americans from low socioeconomic status and help them find better paying jobs. By providing African-American students with the same kinds of educational experiences that enable middle-class white students to acquire skills and attitudes believed to be necessary to achieve success in America was a means to eradicate low socioeconomic status (Pai & Adler). Albeit, civil rights actions and equal educational opportunities were in place (Pai & Adler, 2001), African-American students still are not developing well in these programs remaining culturally deprived throughout their schooling process (Pai & Adler, 2001).

In 2002, the *Elementary and Secondary Education Act of 1965* was amended "To close the achievement gap with accountability, flexibility, and choice, so that no child is left behind" (S. Res. 107, 2001). The aim of the *No Child Left Behind* (NCLB) Act is to ensure that all students receive a meaningful and just opportunity to receive a high quality education and meet the challenging state standards and assessments (NCLB, 2002). Though a large number of successful strategies and philosophies for providing effective learning environments for African—American students were identified, tested, and proven effective (Edelin, 1990), African-American students are still not developing well in the Great Society programs (Pai & Adler, 2001). African-American leadership had no voice in the developmental process of the Great Society programs (Pai & Adler, p. 65).

To ensure that evidence-based strategies be present in the curriculum, according to Edelin (1990), African-American leaders, constituents, and advocates must attend meetings where decisions and policies about educating African-American students are being established. African and African-American leaders always knew how to educate African-American students but the philosophies and teaching strategies that proved to be effective were not present in the public school system because African-American educators were not included in the policy and decision-making process (Edelin, 1990). To provide a real education and meet the distinct needs of African-American students who attend urban public schools, purported Edelin (1990), the first step is to change the negative pathology approach that uses terms such as disadvantaged, permanent underclass, at risk, minority, culturally deprived, and low-achievers to define students (Edelin, 1990; O'Brien, 1998).

Defining students as minority or academically disadvantaged promotes low self-esteem, according to Marks and Tonso (2006) who purported, self-esteem is vital to the academic success of African-American students. Marks and Tonso continued by stating when African-American students learn to believe that they are not capable academically, those thoughts become self-fulfilling prophecies that turn into reality for many students. On the other hand, when African-American students learn to believe that they and their thoughts have value and that they descend from a rich heritage, they too, will want to live out that reality (Marks & Tonso). Without an understanding of history, people cannot be whole and the process of becoming whole must begin by having a clear understanding of World History, including African history (Clarke, 1990).

Discovering and implementing the most appropriate teaching practices, strategies, models, and theories for African-American students who attend urban public schools, are an ongoing struggle yet, critical to the liberation for African and African-American people in the United States (Worrill, 2007). Woodson (1998) stated the following:

> In the absence of an educational system that is culturally relevant, grounded in history, and directed towards some grand future visions for Africans (Thompson, 1995), is a mis-education system that consistently fails to serve the interest of African people both historically and presently. (Rashid, 2005, p. 543)

Culture must be honored while meeting the underlying initiatives requirements of the local, state, and national mandates (Boutte & Strickland, 2008; Olivia, 2005). This approach to the schooling process predicates on the belief that the culture of African descent is important in general but more specifically, important to the well-being of humanity (Carruthers, 1995; Solomon, 1996).

Educators must have a responsibility to infuse indigenous culture specifically, etiquette and nutrition, in the educational experience for African-American female-students who attend urban public schools and help them learn meaningful yet, effective processes of self-preservation, which is the purpose of this book. A plethora of African-American female-youth are not meeting Adequate Yearly Progress (AYP) in public schools (Chicago Public Schools) in that, many African-American female students are failing in public schools in the Chicago land area. In addition, according to ISBE (n.d.) and Chicago Public Schools (n.d.), several public schools in Chicago are closing because the schools are failing our nation's female-youth; "The board gave a ringing endorsement to [Mayor] Emanuel's vision for a downsized school system, which he argues will help combat a massive budget deficit and allow the district to distribute scarce resources more efficiently" (Chicago Tribune, 2013). Closing schools where students are underperforming may or may not provide effective results for students. The way to achieve meaningful yet, effective results for teachers and students are to design curriculum in accord to students' cultural needs and provide learning environments that align with learning objectives.

The Root of the Problem

BEFORE WE WORK to find solutions to the problems our nation's female-youth encounter, we have to acknowledge and understand the root cause. Little research has been conducted regarding the way culture in general and African descendant's culture in particular, is applied to the educational experience for African-American students who attend public schools in Chicago (Davis, 2005). Students must be involved in their schooling processes and be interested in what they are being taught. Yes, the current core subjects that are implemented in curricula like math, science, and social studies are sufficient yet; students need to be excited about their learning, as means for them to want to learn. Educators must find ways to capture and maintain students' attention regarding core subject matter. Why are so many female students failing in Chicago public elementary schools? This means that many of these girls will not graduate on time, if at all, leaving them with less likely of a chance to enter college. The majority of these young girls will drop out of school, get pregnant, and find themselves on governmental assistant programs. As a result, many of these young girls will lose their self-confidence only to find themselves in unruly relationships that oftentimes lead them on negative journeys throughout the remainder of their lives.

Author's Experience

I CAN ATTEST TO the aforementioned, as I have personally experienced those behaviors. I dropped out of high school at the young age of 16, got pregnant, got married, got an annulment two months later, and found myself in abusive relationships for several years before I decided to make a change in my own life. But my issues started way before high school. These misguided behaviors started in elementary school. I was an avid athlete! My sport was volleyball and I thought that I was pretty good too! Having the ability to play the sport gave me confidence and if I could be honest, the main reason why I wanted to attend school at the time. I was bullied in school by many of the girls who did not like me—some people said it was because I was cute and had long hair but who knows. All I know is that I was bullied but maintained focus on my sport. The learning environment at school was fine, I guess but what I was being taught was not so fine. I remember the seventh grade: Several years ago, as a seventh grade student in a social studies class with a classroom student population of about 25 African-American students, culture infusion consisted of learning that Christopher Columbus discovered America and that the African presence began with slavery. This experience was the start of the preconceived ideas that descendants of African history and culture was more authentic than what educators taught in the 1980s. To believe that African-Americans sat around in darkness waiting for Christopher Columbus to show up and flip on the light switch or that slavery was the start of a civilized society for African-Americans, is to ignore the significant contributions that descendants of African people made to the African continent, the United States, and other parts of the world.

I graduated and went to high school with the motivation to continue to play volleyball yet, learned more about myself and the crises that African-American female-youth encounter; I just wanted to get along with everyone. Continuing throughout high school with my studies and playing volleyball, I met a young man who at the time became my high school sweetheart. What a great time that was until my team went to the playoffs, we won of course! But soon after, I learned that I was pregnant but not before I found out I was accepted to attend the University of Columbus in Ohio with a full scholarship. I was so excited but had to make a life changing decision at the young age of 16. I had to inform both my coaches whom were obviously disappointed when they had to tell me that I could no longer play volleyball hence, no scholarship. Not only did that news affect my self-esteem but having to walk around the school pregnant with a big belly was embarrassing so I felt the best thing for me to do, at that time, was to drop out of school. Ten years passed before I decided to do something meaningful with my life. Before then, I had no support group but rather several men who told me only things I wanted to hear, which lead to another pregnancy and several abusive (physical and mental) relationships— my life was very dreadful as a youth but I overcame my obstacles and want our nation's female-youth whom are experiencing personal difficulty to know that they too can overcome and succeed no matter the situation.

The process of overcoming obstacles requires just as much time and energy that one puts into unhealthy relationships, even more. Doing the wrong thing is easy but change, in most cases, is hard to do without a healthy support system and motivation. My inspiration came from my children. I knew that I wanted more for them so I had to do more for myself. After having dropped out of high school in 1987, 10 years later in 1997, I went back to school to obtain my High School Equivalency Certificate otherwise known as GED and never looked back. I went on to earn a Bachelor of Fine Arts degree in 2001 from The Illinois

Institute of Art in Media, Arts, & Animation; my Master of Arts degree in 2004 from Northeastern Illinois University in Inner City Studies; and my Doctorate of Education in Educational Leadership with a Specialization in Curriculum and Instruction, in 2011. I have studied the issues that are deeply embedded within the public education system and I am working to make a meaningful, yet effective change for our nation's female-youth who are not meeting AYP in public schools. A significant relationship exists between culture infusion methods and African-American student achievement.

If African-American female-youth are to be successful in public schools, infusion of indigenous culture in the curriculum is necessary. School leaders should collaborate with educators and curriculum development specialists to determine what is appropriate for students to know and understand about indigenous culture. In addition, ensure the team is educated about authentic African history and culture, design an extensive curriculum plan according to the cultural, educational, social, and emotional needs and interests of attending students, involve students in certain aspects of developing curriculum such as (class activities, field trips, appearance of and classroom environment), then implement the appropriate curriculum in accord to plan. Why are public elementary school teachers failing so many female students? A large number of elementary grade-level female-student failures are a direct result of poor curriculum design and curriculum infusion practices (what and how students are being taught while in school). Students can achieve academic success when curriculum and teaching behaviors align. Curriculum must align with teaching behaviors therefore teachers must learn how to align teaching behaviors with curriculum. Do teachers know whether or not students understand the lesson? Do teachers identify whether students are interested in what they are being taught? Teachers must know for whom they are teaching. Get to know each student and learn what s/he already knows about the subject you, the teacher, are teaching. Develop lesson plans suitable for students learning needs, which offer a better chance of achieving desired learning outcomes from students. Examine the lesson plan to ensure accuracy and verify that it aligns with desired results. "It is impossible to determine if certain teaching behaviors are effective unless we know whether or not students learn as an end result of these teaching behaviors" (Hunt, Touzel, and Wiseman, 1999, p. 3).

Effective Teaching

TEACHERS BEHAVIOR IS associated with student achievement according to researchers who report that attitudes, use of time, organization, communication, focus, feedback monitoring, questioning, pacing, and review and closure all correlate with student achievement (Kauchak and Eggen, 1997, as cited in Hunt, Touzel, and Wiseman, 1999). Effective teaching behaviors are most likely to have a positive effect on student behavioral and performance outcomes.

Attitudes

Many people believe that teachers' attitude play a significant role in student achievement according to Bruning, Schraw, & Ronning (1995) as cited in Hunt, Touzel, and Wiseman (1999), "Teachers who hold the belief that they and their schools indeed do, or can, have an important positive effect on students and their learning are said to have high *teacher efficacy*" (p. 10). Classrooms teachers with high efficacy have a high rate of student achievement and use praise rather than criticism as means for motivation and reward.

Effective Use of Time

High efficacy teachers tend to work well with students who are not meeting AYP, are more accepting of students, never give up on students, and make effective use of their time. Researchers suggest that the more time used during the schooling process on instruction, the higher level of student academic success.

Organization

Teachers should be well organized. Researchers contend that organized teachers have higher achieving students as compared to unorganized teachers (Hunt, Touzel, and Wiseman, 1999). Students can tell whether or not teachers are prepared and organized therefore, teachers should explain the classroom's organizational structure that should include both classroom management and educational management. Organized teachers start class on time with instructional material ready and an established routine for teaching/learning (Hunt, Touzel, and Wiseman, 1999). Organized classroom teachers are good planners and makes sure instructional material aligns with learning objectives and the learning environment is appropriate for attending students.

Communication

Researchers in the field of education have found a positive link between language clarity and student success. Teachers should be very clear when verbally communicating with students to ensure information is transmitted precisely as intended. Teachers should refrain from using ambiguous words and phrases from classroom studies and interactions with students, keep the discourse connected that leads to a goal via a point-by-point planned process, use appropriate transitions leading to the next topic area, and place emphasis on information that students should remember, "If something is of special importance, tell the students" (Hunt, Touzel, and Wiseman, 1999, p.12).

Focus

Capturing and maintaining students' attention to the lesson should be established on the outset of the instructional experience. Students are better connected to the body of the lesson that follows when they are focused on the lesson at the beginning. To avoid difficulties in attention and focus later in the lesson, teachers should establish an effective framework for the lesson and its direction at the beginning, which helps both the teacher and students throughout the learning process (Hunt, Touzel, and Wiseman).

Feedback

Feedback is information that discloses whether or not one is on course, according to Wiggins (1999) who stated, "Feedback is evidence that confirms or disconfirms the correctness of my actions" (p. 134). Teachers who provide feedback to students on a regular basis regarding their school work performance (oral or written) tend to have higher achieving students (Hunt, Touzel, and Wiseman). Feedback motivates students to check the accuracy of their own work and provides a sense of balance in the classroom (Hunt, Touzel, and Wiseman).

Monitoring

Teachers who have the quality of *withitnes* in that, they have been identified as having good monitoring skills are more likely to identify whether or not students are engaged in the classwork, understand the classwork, attentive to the classwork, and able to adjust the teaching behaviors accordingly (Hunt, Touzel, and Wiseman). According to O'Keeefe and Johnson (1987) as cited by Hunt, Touzel, and Wiseman, effective monitoring ability is an important skill that relates to increased student learning. Teachers who display such a skill are more likely to have a positive classroom learning environment. Teachers who have the *withitness* ability are not only aware of what is going on in the classroom but these teachers actually care about their students classroom experiences.

Questioning

Teachers should ask their students questions to learn what students already know about the lesson that is being taught. According to Hunt, Touzel, and Wiseman, different type questions are asked for different learning purposes and depending on the lesson being taught will determine the type of questioning. Teachers should have the ability to ask well-developed questions; a necessary skill for effective teachers. If the lesson is to focus on basic skill attainment then low cognitive questioning is required but if students are required to analyze or evaluate particular subject matter then high cognitive questions should be applied according to Hunt, Touzel, and Wiseman who reported, "Both high and low cognitive questions can correlate positively with student achievement" (p. 14).

Pacing

The amount of subject matter being introduced and the quantity and type of verbal interactions between students and teacher, in this case, is referred to as pacing. Albeit, establishing an appropriate pace could be a difficult skill for teachers to develop, appropriate pacing is associated with student achievement (Hunt, Touzel, and Wiseman). When the lesson is moved at a quick-pace the attention and engagement of students is at a higher rate than lessons that are moved at a slower, more systematic pace. Teachers should be careful not to conduct instruction at too fast of a pace as to decrease the chances of students not comprehending and losing interest in the lesson. Appropriate classroom pacing requires good questioning skills from teachers ((Hunt, Touzel, and Wiseman).

Review and Closure

As means to help improve student academic achievement, according to Hunt, Touzel, and Wiseman, clear review and closure of students' lessons are necessary. Teachers should review either close to the beginning, in the middle, or at the end of each lesson to summarize and help students connect what was learned already to the learning that is to come. Before the end of a lesson, teachers should determine the level of understanding each student has about the particular lesson, which provides closure. Several techniques could be used to ensure closure including but not limited to the following: Use of related questioning, classroom/homework assignments, and general classroom participation/discussion. Following each technique should reveal pertinent information that leads to and introduces the next lesson, which helps students understand and identify how to or where to begin the next lesson (Hunt, Touzel, and Wiseman). Researchers recommend teachers to ask their students to provide, in their own words, points of information to describe the learning that have been covered, as means to ensure that students understand the topic and have a point to build on for the subsequent lesson.

Effective Teacher Qualities

A POSITIVE RELATIONSHIP EXISTS between the characteristics of effective teachers and increasing academic achievement according to researchers who reported seven different effective teacher traits:

1. *Teacher Character Trait*: Effective teachers are enthusiastic, inspiring, positive, compassionate, task-oriented and well-organized, respectful, understanding, flexible, democratic, have high expectations for students, do not seek recognition, do not care about being liked, are able to overcome student stereotypes, have good listening skills, able to express emotions, and takes responsibility for student learning.
2. *What the Teacher Knows*: Effective teachers are experienced in their field of study and have a plethora of factual information.
3. *What the Teacher Teaches*: Effective teachers not only cover criterion for which students are accountable but go beyond to provide maximum content study.
4. *How the Teacher Teaches*: Effective teachers provide clarity and variety, creates and sustain momentum, effectively utilizes small groups, encourages students to participate, observe and devote attention to students, provide structure and effective teaching and learning environments, take advantage of unexpected events, monitor seatwork, ensure that both open-ended and lower-order questions are infused, involves students in peer teaching, allow

large-group discussion/instruction, provide instruction in small amounts to avoid complexity, does not use too much busy work or traditional materials, express to students the importance of what should be learned, explain the thinking processes necessary for learning, and foresee and resolve any misunderstandings.

5. ***What the Teacher Expects***: Effective teachers establish student-expectations, hold students accountable for their actions, and encourage parents to participate in the educational process of students.

6. ***How the Teacher Reacts to Pupils***: Effective teachers are accepting and supportive of students, consistent when dealing with students, make slight yet meaningful use of student criticism, demonstrate with-itness, use praise meaningfully, use incentives, adjust to student stages of development, individualize instructional material, engage students who do not volunteer to participate in class discussion, provide appropriate wait-time for student response to questioning, encourage students, help students by providing immediate feedback, and mindful of and sensitive to different cultural groups and accommodate accordingly.

7. ***How Teachers Manage***: Effective teachers demonstrate proficiency in planning, have strong organizational skills, always on time for class, perform multiple tasks simultaneously, accept some noise in the classroom, have group alerting techniques, persistent in requiring on-time class/homework, reduce classroom disturbances, use mild punishment practices, establish and maintain a peaceful learning environment, and hold students to academic achievement standards (Hunt, Touzel, and Wiseman, p. 15).

Effective teacher characteristics should be demonstrated to students in all learning environments if the aim of educators is to inspire and enlighten students. The aforementioned (**Effective Teaching** and **Effective Teacher Qualities**) are tools that could be used to help improve the quality of education for our nation's youth and should be considered while implementing curriculum. The following you will find information that will inform instructors about an innovative program that is designed to support elementary grade-level female students and motivate them to want to learn. Students have to be interested in what they are learning and the team at SGR belief is that we have developed a program that will meaningfully yet, effectively contribute in this ongoing process of discovering and maintaining student-interests in their schooling processes and finding best methods of improving the quality of education for female youth.

SGR: An All-Girl Youth Program

THE SGR PROGRAM is comprised with curriculum content that tailors toward the cultural interests of African-American female-youth. Information within the body of this book should be used to equip educators with meaningful, yet effective teaching strategies that, when implemented appropriately, will work to help improve persona; the quality of education; and AYP for African-American female students who attend public schools. Throughout the body of this work is the curriculum for the program therefore; teachers should find best methods of infusing the SGR curriculum into the educational process in that, discovering best teaching practices (classwork, homework, activities, instruction, lessons etc.) that will ensure that students will be able to understand the objectives and attain the learning goals. For assistance with developing instructional material and other SGR educational activities, visit our website.

Philosophy

SGR LEADERS WORK to bring pride with prospects of students bringing pride to SGR. The belief is that students will begin at an early age to discover a sense of purpose in life that fosters dignity and achievement as well as grow to respect themselves, each other, and the community. Mentors will work to understand and cultivate the various kinds of intelligences such as social, emotional, intellectual, and character. Through hands-on activities and mentor guidance, SGR leaders will work to enable students to make discoveries about themselves, their community, humanity, and the world. SGR leaders believe that guided learning will engage both individuals and groups. Educators at SGR will help enable students to become fulfilled persons, respectful community members, and meaningful yet, effective participants in a rapidly changing world.

The team at SGR believes that schooling is about providing opportunities of learning that tailor toward the cultural interests of attending students. Education at SGR is also about schooling for all, as educators must learn how each student learns, as a means to implement appropriate teaching behaviors that will work to bring about desired learning outcomes. The focus and specific interests of SGR are the enlightening and empowerment of all students, their families, neighborhoods, and the total development and growth of all nations. It is the firm belief of the team at SGR that students want to learn and capable yet, students are more inclined to *want* to learn when they are interested in what they are being taught, have an appropriate learning environment, and have a compassionate support group throughout their learning experience. SGR offers a mentorship program that works to enlighten, guide, and support students throughout the SGR journey of learning.

Mission Statement

Our mission is to empower female youth who are underperforming (not meeting AYP standards) in their schools' general education classrooms by providing appropriate learning environments and infusing specialized educational programs in the curriculum that will work to enable dynamic behavioral skills, as a means to help girls thrive in the SGR program, their general education classroom, at home, and the global society.

Vision Statement

Leaders at SGR will work to help improve the quality of education for female youth who attend public schools. SGR will partner with parents and the community to provide a meaningful yet, effective learning environment for all attending students. By infusing the curriculum with nutritional significance and etiquette coaching that aligns with the cultural interests and needs of attending students, the team at SGR belief is that students will attain self-confidence and educational excellence. Upon successful completion of the program, students will perform more proficiently in their general education classrooms, improve academic and social skills, attain a positive self-image, and understand the relationship between healthy eating habits and a healthy body—inside and out.

Learning Standards Framework for Etiquette & Nutrition

LEARNING STANDARDS ARE statements that define what knowledge and skills students enrolled in the SGR program are expected to know and be able to do. The SGR program standards framework for this phase is divided into two learning areas:

- Etiquette
- Nutrition

Each learning area contains an introduction to the learning area explaining the structure of learning and background information; learning standard; chart of goals, and learning benchmark that define the knowledge and skills for the learning area.

Goals: Broad statements of knowledge and skills that organize the subject matter of the learning area. Each goal contains an explanation of why it is important and how it relates to life beyond school.

Learning Standards: Are content standards that define *what* girls ages 8 to 13 should know and be able to do in the SGR program. Each content standard includes three benchmarks that describe what female youth should know and be able to do.

Learning Benchmarks: Are progress indicators that help gauge students' achievement of each transition standard forming the basis for measuring student achievement over time. The benchmarks build in complexity and rigor from one level to the next, to ensure students have a clear understanding of anticipated learning and learning outcomes.

Performance Standards: The knowledge and skills that students are to perform at various stages of educational development.

Vision for Etiquette Performance

K NOWLEDGE AND UNDERSTANDING of proper etiquette places students in position to recognize the importance of personal values and respect for others are essential to the well-being of all citizens in a global society. Obtaining such qualities will help students lead a pleasant lifestyle that ultimately, progresses into meaningful yet, effective livelihood experiences.

Etiquette Learning Standards

Goal 1: Cultivate polite behavior, as means to attain educational and personal achievement and contribute to building up worthy experiences.

> **Why this goal is important:** *Edelin (1990) asserted, "The African American group lacks cultural integrity, and has started a process of self-correction and consensus-building for the explicit purpose of rectifying this very serious problem" (p.39). Managing behavior fosters integrity.*

Learning Standard:

A. Identify and manage one's attitude.

Session 1	Session 2	Session 3
1. A.1a. Recognize and accurately label attitudes and explain how they are connected to behavior.	1. A.2a. Demonstrate control of attitude in adverse situations and exhibit appropriate manners in social environments.	1. A.3a Analyze how attitudes affect the process of decision-making and appropriate behavior.
1. A.1b. Describe a variety of attitudes and the circumstances that may cause them.	1. A.2b Describe and demonstrate ways to conduct appropriate manners at school, at home, and in other social environments (use scenarios)	1. A.3b Apply strategies to manage behavior and to inspire polite attitudes (use scenarios/role play)

Goal 2: Develop and retain self-respect and respect for others to establish and maintain positive demeanor and relationships.

Why this goal is important: *The most significant contribution one could make to society is respect. One should always pay high or special regard for others, as means to receive high or special regard and promote social generosity.*

Learning Standard:

B. Examine what it means to demonstrate, value, and cultivate respect.

Session 1	Session 2	Session 3
2. B.1a. Recognize how respect is conducted with focus on one's self and interaction with others.	2. B.2a. Describe the significance of self-respect and respect amongst individuals in social environments.	2. B.3a. Analyze the process of applying respect in unfavorable situations (use scenarios/role play).
2. B.1b. Demonstrate respectability (work in groups/role play)	2. B.2b. Express one's current/desired states of the portrayal of respect (use scenarios/provide examples of real life experiences). Set goals to reach desired state of respectability.	2. B.3b. Apply one's desired state of respectability to undesirable situations (use scenarios/role play). Report the outcomes.

Goal 3: Use personal awareness skills to establish the importance of good hygiene.

> **Why this goal is important:** *"Personal hygiene should be practiced not only to keep you healthy, but also to keep others who come into contact with you healthy" (Covelli, 2010).*

Learning Standard:

> C. Enhance and promote self-assured, hygiene behaviors.

Session 1	Session 2	Session 3
3. C.1a. Examine personal hygienic methods (brainstorm; write what comes to mind and discuss with group).	3. C.2a. Explain the importance of personal cleanliness at home and in social environments.	3. C.3a. Explore the various type of female hygiene products and describe best practices as well as appropriate usage(s) for each (e.g., deodorant prevents underarm odor; toothpaste help fight against tooth decay).
3. C.1b. Explain empirical discoveries about hygiene in various situations (teachers learn student's hygiene practices).	3. C.2b. Establish an association with self-assured hygiene behaviors and peer interaction and vice versa (use positive and negative examples—lax in hygiene and peer interaction).	3. C.3b. Prepare a daily personal hygiene regimen include days when not feeling self-assured at home and in social environments.

Goal 4: Demonstrate nurture and care for one-self with focus on hair, nails, and skin in personal, school, and social environments.

Why this goal is important: *Not only should people look good and feel good about their appearances, people should also feel good on the inside, which reflects outwardly in appearance, emotions, and behavior.*

Learning Standard:

D. Explore the basic personal practices of taking care of hair, nails, and skin, as it relates to tact and well-being.

Session 1	Session 2	Session 3
4. D.1a. Explore several issues that could affect the skin.	4. D.2a. Recognize terms and examine the processes of performing a natural manicure and pedicure (fingernail care).	4. D.3a. Explore one's own personal references of hair ideals and practices.
4. D.1b. Express ways that may work to protect the skin and keep it healthy and calm.	4. D.2b. Define related terms and demonstrate step-by-steps process to care for nails.	4. D.3b. Explain the process upkeep of one's everyday hair care including products used (practice using models—mannequins).

Vision for Nutrition Performance

AWARENESS OF DAILY consumption of foods and the affects that certain foods have on the body are significant factors to the livelihood experience. Knowledge and intake of healthy food and nutrients needed to maintain a healthy body will not only nurture the physical aspects of the body and provide good health benefits but will also nurture the mind enabling students to maintain focus in the classroom and enable positive evaluations.

Nutrition Learning Standards

Goal 1: Understand nutrition with emphasis on agriculture (practical course)

> **Why this goal is important:** *"Food is about agriculture, about ecology, about man's relationship with nature, about the climate, about nation-building, cultural struggles, friends and enemies, alliances, wars, [and] religion"* Kurlansky's quotation *(as cited in The National Geographic Society, 2008, p. 29).*

Learning Standard:

> A. Understand the processes of planting, nurturing, growing, and harvesting fruits and vegetables.

Session 1	Session 2	Session 3
1. A.1a. Identify various types of seeds and methods required for sowing nutriments.	1. A.2a. Demonstrate reviewed horticultural techniques.	1. A.3a. Analyze the nutritional values of harvested fruits and vegetables.
1. A.1b. Explain the process of cultivating fruit and vegetables.	4. B.2b. Throughout the process, describe the stages of growth and development of fruit and vegetables (images).	1. A.3b. Illustrate the process of preserving crop during Winter months.

Goal 2: Understand nutrition with emphasis on healthy diet

Why this goal is important: *Jamie Oliver stated, "In fact, research shows that good nutrition and physical activity habits positively affect academic achievement and test scores" (2012).*

Learning Standard:

B. Recognize the essential food groups and nutritional amounts to eat each day.

Session 1	Session 2	Session 3
2. B.1a. Name the food groups that provide specific nutrients needed for a healthy diet (include examples of a variety of foods).	2. B.2a. Describe what counts as one serving from each food group (e.g., ¾ cup fruit juice = 1 serving from the Fruit Group).	2. B.3a. Explain the various ways one could determine the nutritional amounts of food to consume daily (e.g., 14-year-old girl who is tall, and a cheerleader-what should be her calorie intake; plan her lunch).

2. B.1b. From each food group, identify the number of servings that should be consumed each day and name them (plan healthy meals).	2. B.2b. Determine the nutritional daily intake and determine the amounts in calories for women and older adults; kids, teen girls, active women, and most men; and teen boys and active men.	2. B.3b. Plan healthy meals for breakfast, lunch, dinner using all food groups using the standard daily intake for people including, those with lower, average, and higher calorie needs (written, drawings or props, presentation.

From the curriculum, teachers must develop instruction and have class participation to help students understand each learning standard and meet/exceed each goal. In addition, teachers must explain to students why each goal is important. Albeit, each learning area reveals the learning standards and goals, they also explain why each goal is important and must be explained to students as part of the academic learning experience. One statement regarding why each goal is important is stated in each learning standard. However, teachers may choose to provide more examples as to explain why each goal is important. Ensure that each new example provided is based on evidence in the field of study as well as experience. For more information on developing instruction visit our website.

SGR Learning Environment

"Effective learning environments begin with the highest expectations and vision of what our group and our children can be; they involve parents, families, and the community intimately in their work; they are cooperative rather than competitive settings; and they utilize cultural studies, and hands-on, inquiry-based formats" (Edelin, 1990, p.42).

(Curriculum, Environment, & Education Alignment)

STUDENTS BEING THE main client in any educational environment, educators must ensure that curriculum, the classroom environment, and the schooling process all align with the interests of attending student's cultural needs. Students will help design, organize, and maintain their learning environment. Having been small children, being in their presence, and having experience, the leaders at SGR have determined that the learning environment for the etiquette and nutrition program should encompass the following components:

Inner Grounds

* Earthy, Serene Environment
* Infused with Students Colorful Artwork
* Waterfalls
* Plants and Flowers
* Birds & Fish-tanks
* Classrooms & Office Space
* Dining Area & Kitchen
* Restrooms
* Library/Learning Center
* Peace Room
* Vending Machines (all natural & organic)

Outer Grounds

* Garden/Green House
* Parking Lot
* Storage Space
* Play Ground

Students will be involved with the design and upkeep of their learning environment. All Students will have an opportunity to have their works of art displayed. Artwork will be randomly selected, displayed on the walls then rotated to ensure all students have an opportunity to reveal their personal, creative works. In addition, each student will play a role in the maintenance of their learning environment, as means to teach responsibility. Educators will determine best methods to ensure that duties are distributed fair and equally amongst girls, as means to instill effective cohort working, skill development, and organization. Given feminine nature, it seems the female species are extremely sensitive and require essentials on a regular basis. Provided appropriate teaching and learning strategies, enriching cultural environments, and effective teachers that possess meaningful yet, effective teacher characteristics; our nation's female youth will not only thrive in their general education classrooms, the SGR program, at home, and the global society they will also discover age-appropriate behaviorisms, hygienic, and characteristics of female norms.

The Process

THE *SGR ON Saturday's* program will be held at each school that meets the standards if the principal is interested in the program. SGR on Saturdays is a nonprofit, Saturday school program whereby students will meet at their school each Saturday at a specific time. The principal will submit the names and complete a recommendation form for 12 (no more than 14) female students—three students from grade-levels 3rd, 4th, 5th, and 6th who are not meeting AYP and interested in the SGR Saturday program. Classroom teachers and a parent/guardian must approve by signing the appropriate document. Once qualifying students are selected a consultant from the SGR program will visit the school, meet with the principal and arrange to meet with each student individually along with her parent. Parents are required read and sign the program's registration form and guidelines. Upon enrollment, each student will complete an entrance survey and an exit survey at the end of the program. Other ancillary forms such as *Parent Release Forms, Field Trip Approval Forms,* and other will need to be complete and signed by parents at appropriate times (before picture/video days and field trips etc.) otherwise students will not be included in the activity—forms will be handed to parents a week prior to each event. The final step is the interview process. The leaders at SGR want to be sure that selected girls are interested in attending the program therefore we schedule an interview at the school with each girl and her parent or guardian to ensure everyone's approval.

Scope of SGR on Saturday's

The classroom environment should consist of 12 girls no more than 14 total students in a session. The program should run for 12 consecutive Saturdays, for 5 ½ hours, totaling 66 hours. Upon completion, students will have a commencement ceremony honoring their achievements. The school principal must provide appropriate classroom learning areas for the group and outdoor space for gardening. In addition, the principal must agree to the terms that allows for making necessary changes to the classroom environment that aligns with SGR curriculum and learning standards—see above: (*Curriculum, Environment, & Education Alignment*).

A SGR instructor and assistant(s) meet at the participating school each Saturday for 12 consecutive Saturdays. SGR members and students utilize the garden area and classroom(s) designated for the SGR program. The schedule and class structural breakdown as follows:

Saturday's	10:30am-	4:00pm	12weeks
Lunch 45 min.	3/5 min. breaks	Total: 5 ½ hours	

Minutes for Teaching the School Girls Rock (SGR) on Saturday Program

	Etiquette					Nutrition	
Schedule	Behavior	Respect	Hygiene	Upkeep	Schedule	Agriculture	Diet
Sat. 1	90 min.	90 min.			Sat. 1	90 min.	
Sat. 2	90 min.	90 min.			Sat. 2	90 min.	
Sat. 3: Quiz	90 min.	90 min.			Sat. 3	90 min.	
Sat. 4			90 min.	90 min.	Sat. 4		90 min.
Sat. 5			90 min.	90 min.	Sat. 5	.	90 min.
Sat. 6: Quiz		.	90 min.	90 min.	Sat. 6		90 min.
Sat. 7	Role Play	Role Play	Practical	Practical	Sat. 7	Hands-on	Project
Sat. 8	45 min.	45 min.	45 min.	45 min.	Sat. 8	Hands-on	Project

Sat. 9 Quiz	45 min	45 min.	45 min.	45 min.	Sat. 9	Hands-on	Project
Sat. 10	45 min.	45 min.	45 min.	45 min.	Sat. 10	45 min	45 min.
Sat. 11	45 min	45 min	45 min	45 min	Sat. 11	45 min.	45 min.
Sat 12	Final Project				Sat. 12	Final Project	

At the end of the program, each student receives a certificate and the school receives a plaque.

Professional Development Workshop (PDW)

The PDW is designed to provide teachers with necessary tools to assist with implementing the SGR curriculum. School principals who are **not** interested in participating in the *SGR on Saturday* program with SGR instructors, can still implement the SGR program in their school. The first step is to acquire the book: School Girls Rock: Curriculum and Guide to Educational Achievement. Throughout the body of this text will reveal necessary information to assist teachers who are interested in implementing the SGR program at their school. The next step is for the principal to arrange an appointment for an agent from the SGR program to conduct a workshop at his or her school. Upon successful completion of the PDW, educators will have gained skills that will enable them to implement effectively, the SGR program. In addition, each teacher will receive a certificate of completion and the school will be recognized as being participants of the SGR program.

Consultation

The SGR on Saturday's program will end at each school after 12 consecutive sessions conducted by SGR instructors. Throughout the body of this text will reveal necessary information to assist teachers who are interested in implementing the SGR program at their school. SGR consultations are designed for schools that have already launched the SGR program in their schools. *Schools girls* are currently enrolled or have completed the SGR program, these schools are already equipped with the SGR learning environment including the garden, necessary forms, and guidelines. Consultants will be available to assist teachers when necessary to provide additional assistance. Please contact us by phone or visit our website to make an appointment and we will schedule a convenient time to service your addition SGR needs.

We want all *school girls* to be empowered! The SGR program is a meaningful yet, effective program and should be a part of the general education curriculum in all public schools. To continue the efforts from the Saturday school program and maintain continuum, educators can always invite a representative from the SGR program to come and assist, as the SGR program should be an ongoing effort for other girls, particularly girls who are not meeting the AYP standards in attending schools.

The Final Step

Once all pertinent forms have been completed, signed, and returned to the school principal and a SGR agent, the final step to the **Process** is to interview the student. Albeit, each student is referred by the school principal and approved by the parent/ guardian, and classroom teacher, the student is the main client. The purpose of the interview is to ensure that each student is interested in attending the SGR program. The student will be asked a series of questions. If the SGR agent determines that the student is interested in attending the SGR on Saturday's program, the student will be provided with our code of conduct pamphlet and an *entrance survey*. The entrance survey can be found on our website and within the SGR manuscript. The purpose of the entrance survey is to determine what the student already knows and understand about the SGR learning areas. Upon completion of the SGR on Saturday program, students will be issued an *exit survey*. The exit survey contains the same questions provided in the entrance survey. The purpose of the exit survey is to determine whether or not teaching behaviors are effective in that, students learn as an end result. Researchers contend that "The new teacher education programs envision the professional teacher as one who learns from teaching rather than as one who has finished learning how to teach" (Darling-Hammond, 1998, p. 7).

The leaders at SGR have set forth specific learning outcomes for attending students and contingent upon the results of the exit survey and student's behavior as well as other evaluations provided throughout the course of the program will determine if SGR teaching behaviors are effective. All students can learn. To ensure that each student reach set goals, SGR leaders will learn how each student learns, as means to appropriately implement instruction. Leaders will work closely with each student; get to know the various learning styles, plan then apply instruction. Eisner (2004) asserted the following, "In a democracy, the last thing we need is a one-size-fits-all curriculum with one single set of goals for everyone" (p. 8). Discovering and implementing the most appropriate teaching strategies align with the SGR structure.

Effective Instructional Strategies

TEACHERS MIGHT USE several strategies to ensure students learn from teaching behaviors. SGR leaders have analyzed *direct strate*gies and *evidence-based* theories. Depending on the learning environment and learning style(s) of each student will determine the most effective strategies to implement as means to acquire desired learning outcomes. Direct strategies "are those instructional methods that are designed to allow teachers to organize and present material to students in the form in which the students are expected to learn" (Hunt, Touzel, and Wiseman, 1999, p. 117). In short, direct teaching is meaningful yet, effective instruction, according to Hunt, Touzel, and Wiseman (1999), that is used to communicate information or demonstrate skills. How students meet set goals is contingent upon the ways in which teachers design and implement instruction. Utilizing direct strategies are most effective in that, teachers present information; students respond by applying knowledge or practice a skill then teachers provide feedback (Hunt, Touzel, and Wiseman). Researchers provide four commonly used methods to directly transmit information to students:

1. Lecture—Oral presentation. Tell students what you wish for them to know. Example: Explain what it means to have a pleasant attitude.
2. Demonstration—Visual presentation. Show students what you want them to learn. Example: Show happy facial expressions. Set up scenarios in the classroom that indicates pleasant, social conduct.

3. Drill—Repeat the objective after students have demonstrated their understanding. Drill provides an opportunity for students to practice and receive feedback. When students understand the objectives by demonstrating through drill and receiving feedback, they are more likely to retain information longer and completely.
4. Teacher-led-discussion—Have open-ended questions with students who want to participate. Request class participation. This strategy enables students to connect their personal experience and provokes interests in the discussion.

Effective teachers should utilize a variety of strategies to determine the most appropriate tactic(s) to implement in the given learning environment (Hunt, Touzel, and Wiseman) and in accord with student readiness. Researchers maintain that "students cannot transfer skills they do not possess" so teachers must ensure that students demonstrate the readiness characteristics necessary to perform a given task, which can be accomplished by assessing the extent to which students can perform assigned tasks (Friedman, Harwell, and Schnepel, 2006, p. 91).

Approach: SGR Curriculum

THE TWO LEARNING areas in the SGR program include *Etiquette* and *Nutrition*. Each learning area contains learning standards and desired learning outcomes. Below are some tips and examples of how to approach the SGR learning standards that teachers might use to help determine student's readiness levels, as means to ensure all students reach desired performance outcomes. One learning standard for the etiquette learning area is to *identify and manage one's attitude*. Session 1, at the end of the course students should be able to *recognize and accurately label attitudes and explain how they are connected to behavior*. When teaching about attitude, teachers should begin the learning process by asking each student to write down everything s/he knows about attitude. Then ask students to get together in small groups of 3 or 4 students to share their lists. Finally, the teacher should write student's responses on the chalk board exactly how they present them.

	Stage 1	Stage 2	Stage 3
Individual Task	Write down what you know about attitude	Look at what you have come up with and think about how they connect to behavior	Provide one article to each group about attitudes/ behavior. Read together in a group then write a group report to prepare in class
Small Groups (3-4)	Share and discuss list with peers	Get together in your group to discuss ideas	Get together in your group to assign/ discuss task
Whole Group	What did students come up with/ teacher writes their answers on the chalk board	What did students come up with/ teacher writes their answers on the chalk board	Groups are given time to work on report. Start a new lesson plan at Stage 1 on how to write a report

Stage 1 = Using new knowledge. Stage 2 = Experimental practice.
Stage 3 = Further practice.

Educators may find the abovementioned instructional methods of infusing SGR objectives in the schooling process a meaningful yet, effective teaching strategy, which can be used to implement each SGR learning area. The above chart/learning theory was created by Rita Smilkstein, adopted by SGR leaders then tailored to meet the SGR learning standards.

Recommendations

APPROPRIATE GOVERNMENT AGENCIES, CPS, ISBE and all constituents should work together and designate etiquette education and nutrition education as core academic subjects. Community leaders, principals, teachers, parents, and others should not assume that all female-youth understand or even practice appropriate etiquette and nutrition behaviors. There is a relationship between what one eats and how one behaves, which has an effect on the value of one's livelihood. It is the duty of educators to provide the best educational programs and learning environments for our nation's female-youth, if our aim is to uplift them, empower them, and provide them with meaningful yet, effective cultural experiences that will enable them to become successful in their personal and professional lives. When the SGR program is implemented effectively, female-youth as well as educators will thrive. I am confident the SGR program will change the current state of behavior and help improve test scores of female-youth who are underperforming in public school learning environments.

Summary and Conclusion

IN THE YEAR 2013, the majority of our nation's female youth who attend public schools, particularly African-American female youth in Chicago, are still performing below the local, state, and national mandates—students are failing and after decades, educators are still trying to find best suited teaching methods. While working to meet the abovementioned mandates, researchers assert that culture must be honored; culture is important to the well-being of humanity. The ultimate purpose of the SGR program is to empower our nation's female youth and motivate them to want to learn by offering a meaningful yet, effective learning environment that tailors toward the cultural interests of attending students. Providing students with a nurturing learning environment that fosters gardening and etiquette education may help each student build upon a healthy eating lifestyle and personal value system, "The primary aim of education is to enable youngsters to learn how to invent themselves—to learn how to create their own minds" (Eisner, 2004, p. 10).

Recommendations invite stakeholders and all constituents to participate in authorizing the SGR program to be a part of the schooling process for students who are not meeting AYP standards in public schools, particularly in Chicago. With support from community leaders; principals; teachers; and parents, we can work collectively to help improve the quality of education for attending students in public schools. Criteria for starting a SGR program at your school:

1. Recommend a school/students
2. Complete necessary forms
3. Submit other required documents
4. Saturday school availability
5. Classroom and garden accessibility

The SGR program leaders tailor specialized educational services toward female youth who are not meeting the AYP in public schools. We use evidence-based information from the field of education to develop specialized programs that will work to improve student readiness and AYP scores. Students are capable of learning and attaining academic success yet, students are more apt to learn when they are interested in what they are being taught. We encourage female youth to believe in their dreams and work hard to make them come true. The SGR program leaders will work to effectively design and provide a variety of specialized programs for our nation's youth, particularly for young girls who are underperforming in public schools. Etiquettes and Nutrition is the first set of courses yet, several others will follow including but not limited to:

- African/Language Arts
- Creative Art
- Athletics
- Ethics
- Social and Emotional
- Anti-bullying

All forms can be downloaded from our website. For more information and to learn more about other services including costs and fees, please visit our website *www.shadavali.com* or call 773.634.8383.

References

Boutte, G., & Strickland, J. (2008). Making African-American culture and history central to early childhood teaching and learning. *The Journal of Negro Education. 77*(2), 131-142

Dewey, J. (1997). Experience and Education: The Kappa Delta Pi Lecture Series. New York, NY: Simon & Schuster, Carruthers, J. (1995). African-centered education. *An African Worldview*, 2(7), 1-3. Retrieved, June 16, 2008 from *http://www.africawithin.com/carruthers/african education.htm*

Chicago Public Schools (n.d.). Retrieved March 1, 2004 from: *http://www.cps.edu/Programs/Academic_and_enrichment/Pages/Academic.aspx*

Davis, P. (2005). The origins of African American culture and its significance in African American student academic success. *Journal of Thought, 40*(1), 43-59.

Edelin, R. (1990). Curriculum and Cultural identity: In the *Infusion of African and African American Content in the School Curriculum: Proceedings of the First National Conference* 1989. Morristown: Aaron Press.

Eisner, E. (2004). Preparing for today and tomorrow. *Educational Leadership, 61(4),* 6-10.

Friedman, M., Harwell, D., & Schnepel, K. (2006). Effective instruction: A Handbook of evidence-based strategies. Columbia, SC. The Institute for Evidence-Based Decision-Making in Education, Inc.

Hammond-Darling, L. (1998). Teacher learning that supports student learning. *Educational Leadership,* 6-11.

Hunt, G., Touzel, T., & Wiseman, D. (1999). Effective teaching: Preparation and implementation. (3rd ed.). Springfield, IL. Charles C. Thomas Publisher, Ltd.

Illinois State Board of Education. (n.d.). Retrieved September 16, 2004 from: http://www.isbe.net/ils/pdf/ils_introduction.pdf

Marks, J., & Tonso, K. (2006). African-centered education: An approach to schooling for social justice for African American students. *Education, 126(3),* 481-494.

Merriam-Webster. (Inc.). (2005). *The Merriam-Webster Collegiate Dictionary (11th ed.).* United States: Library of Congress.

Nobles, W. (1990). The Infusion of African and African American Content: A question of content and intent. In the Infusion of African and African American Content in the School Curriculum: Proceedings of the first national conference 1989. Morristown: Aaron Press.

No Child Left Behind Act of 2001 (2002). Retrieved June 14, 2007 from: http://www.ed.gov/policy/elsec/leg/esea02/index.html?exp=0

Oliver, J. (n.d). Retrieved October 19, 2012, from: http://www.actionforhealthykids.org/

Olivia, P. (2005). Developing the curriculum (6th ed.). Boston: Allyn and Bacon.

Pai, Y., & Adler, S. (2001). Cultural foundations of education (3rd ed.). Upper Saddle River, New Jersey: Merrill Prentice Hall.

Rashid, K. (2005). Slavery of the mind: Carter G. Woodson and Jacob H. Carruthers—Intergenerational discourse on African education and social change. *Western Journal of Black Studies, 29*(1), 542.

Shujaa, M. (1996). Beyond desegregation: The politics of quality in African American schooling. Thousand Oaks, California: Corwin Press.

Shujaa, M. (1998). Too much schooling too little education: A paradox of black life in white societies. Trenton NJ: Africa World Press.

Smilkstein, R. (2003). We're born to learn: Using the brain's natural learning process to create today's curriculum. Thousand Oaks, California: Corwin Press, Inc.

Solomon, I. (1996). Workshops on a multicultural curriculum: Issues and caveats. *Education, 117*(1), 81-84.

S. Res. 107, Cong., 115 Cong. Rec. 1425 (2002) (enacted).

The National Geographic Society. (2008). Edible: An Illustrated Guide to the World's Food Plants.

Wiggins, G. (1999). Assessing student performance: Exploring the purpose and limits of testing. San Francisco, CA: John Wiley & Sons, Inc.

Woodson, C. (1998). The mis-education of the Negro. Trenton, NJ: Africa World Press, Inc.

Worrill, C. (2007). Implementing an African-centered curriculum in schools. *Chicago Defender, 102*(59), 8.

Registration Information

All Registration Forms Can be Downloaded from our Website

The entrance/exit survey tool should be given to each student upon entering the SGR program and again upon completion.

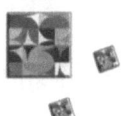

SGR: Entrance/Exit Survey. **Date** _____.

1. Name: Birthday: Phone#:

2. Do you know what etiquette means? Please circle: Yes or No.

3. In your own words, what does etiquette mean to you?

    _____.

4. In thinking about etiquette, do the words behavior; respect; hygiene; and upkeep enter your mind? Please circle: Yes or No. In a few words, please explain.

    _____.

5. Do you believe you practice proper etiquette every day? Circle: Yes or No?

6. Do you know what agriculture means? Please circle: Yes or No.

7. In your own words, what does horticulture mean to you?

   _____.

   _____.

8. In thinking about horticulture, do the words agriculture and nutrition enter your mind? Please circle: Yes or No.

9. Do you nurture your mind and body with healthy practices? Circle: Y or N.

10. Would you like to learn/share the SGR program? Please circle: Yes or No.

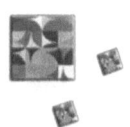

SCHOOL GIRLS ROCK
PO BOX 53310, CHICAGO, IL 60653
PHONE: (773) 624.8383 | *WWW.SHADAVALI.COM*
RECOMMENDATION FORM—PREQUALIFICATION

Principal and classroom teacher(s)

We are excited about the School Girls Rock program (SGR)! The start of classes brings for all of us a mix of new experiences, familiar classmates, and new friends. We are pleased to service your school, excited about meeting your students, and looking forward to getting acquainted with you and your teachers. Please answer the following questions, sign, and return this document to me by _____, 2013.

Name of Principal: _____

Name of School: _____

1. Please provide the names and grade-levels of 12 no more than 14 students who you recommend that qualifies and interested in attending the SGR program (For more space, attach additional sheets of this size):

2. Do the above mentioned students know about the SGR program? Is so, please explain how they learned about the program and tell us if all are interested in learning more and enrolling. If not, please inform them by sharing our handout and other pertinent SGR information. (For more space, attach additional sheets of this size):

3. Of the 12—14 students you recommend, have you informed the parent/guardian about your recommendation and students interests in the SGR program? Is yes, please provide his/her contact information (best phone number to be reached and email) of the parent/guardian of each student you have listed above. (For more space, attach additional sheets of this size):

4. How do believe the above mentioned students you recommended qualify for the SGR program? (For more space, attach additional sheets of this size):

5. To qualify for enrollment in the SGR program each student must be a 3rd, 4th, 5th, and 6th grade, female-youth in attendance at your school and does not meet the Adequate Yearly Progress (AYP). Are the above listed names all female students? Circle one: Yes or No. Are all female students in 3rd, 4th, 5th, or sixth grade? Circle one: Yes or No

6. Are the above mentioned students meeting AYP in current school-year? Circle one: Yes or No. What is the average AYP for the names listed above?

7. Attach a copy of your School Improvement Plan for Advancing Academic Achievement (SIPAAA) for the current school-year—the "AYP" segment of the SIPAAA report is sufficient.

We look forward to assisting with improving the quality of learning behaviors for our nation's female youth—one school at a time!

RECOMMENDATION FORM—PREQUALIFICATION FORM CONTINUED

For each student the principal recommends, the following document should be signed and dated by both the principal and teacher then submitted to SGR.

Principal Information

I, principal _____ of (name of school) _____ will recommend (student name) _____ Grade: _____ room: _____ to the SGR program. (Student name) _____ Classroom teacher's name is _____.

Principal's signature: _____

Date: _____

Classroom Teacher Information

I, classroom teacher _____ agree with the principal's recommendation for (student) _____ Grade: ____ room: ____ to enroll in the SGR program. (Student name) _____ is interested in the SGR program (circle one) **Yes No Not sure**. Classroom teacher's signature: _____

Date: _____

At (name of your school) _____, we have a classroom(s) available to accommodate the SGR learning environment. Circle one: **Yes, we have *accommodations*. Not at this time.**

Please note: All schools must provide an appropriate learning environment to accommodate the SGR program: Classroom and an outdoor garden (indoor green house is acceptable).

Please be sure to Attach Accommodating Documents along with your Recommendation Forms and SIPAAA.

Please check here ____ and initial here ____ that you have attached the SIPAAA for the current school year.

Please provide your contact information.

Name: _____

Email: _____

Telephone: _____

We look forward to School Girls Rock on Saturday's at your School too!

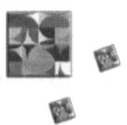

Parent Release Form for Media Recording

I, the undersigned, do hereby grant or deny permission to School Girls Rock (SGR) to use the image of my child, _____, as marked by my selection(s) below. Such use includes the display, distribution, publication, transmission, or otherwise use of photographs, images, and/or video taken of my child for use in materials that include, but may not be limited to, printed materials such as brochures and newsletters, videos, and digital images such as those on the our website.

❑ Deny permission to use my child's image at all.

❑ Grant permission to use my child's image in the following ways (mark all that apply):

   ❑ **Limited usage:** I want my child's image used *within* the SGR setting only (not in the larger community of ShaDavAli Multimedia Studio, Inc.).

   ❑ **Limited usage:** I want my child's image used for *educational* materials only (not marketing). This could be either within SGR or in the larger community. One example of this could be videos in parent education classes.

   ❑ **Limited usage:** I want my child's image used on *printed* materials only (no digital or video use).

❑ **Unrestricted usage:** I give unrestricted permission for my child's image to be used in print, video, and digital media. I agree that these images may be used by SGR and the larger community of ShaDavAli Multimedia Studio, Inc., for a variety of purposes and that these images may be used without further notifying me.

Parent/guardian signature: _____

Date: _____

Please make a copy of applicable form(s) for your records then submit original to a SGR agent. Or, mail/email to:

Dr. Andrea Green-Gibson
PO Box 53310: Chicago, IL. 60653
shadavali@gmail.com
www.shadavali.com

Thank you for finding interest in the SGR program! :*)

Andrea Green-Gibson, Ed.D
Founder, School Girls Rock
CEO, ShaDavAli Multimedia Studio, Inc.

www.ingramcontent.com/pod-product-compliance
Lightning Source LLC
Chambersburg PA
CBHW030524290526
45786CB00004B/1612